Understandin

OSTEOPOROSIS

Dr Juliet E. Compston

Published by Family Doctor Publications Limited
in association with the British Medical Association

© Family Doctor Publications 1998
Reprinted 1999

Medical Editor: Dr Tony Smith
Consultant Editor: Maria Stasiak
Cover Artist: Colette Blanchard
Medical Artist: Philip Wilson
Design: MPG Design, Blandford Forum, Dorset
Printing: Reflex Litho, Thetford, Norfolk, using acid-free paper

ISBN: 1-898205-24-8

Contents

Introduction 1

How does osteoporosis develop? 4

Who develops osteoporosis? 10

Symptoms and signs of osteoporosis 15

Diagnosis of osteoporosis 22

Treatment of osteoporosis: general measures 28

Self-help measures 33

Drugs used in treatment of osteoporosis: HRT 40

Non-HRT treatments of osteoporosis 50

Treatment of less common forms of osteoporosis 61

Questions and answers 64

Glossary 66

Useful addresses 68

Index 69

Introduction

We are all familiar with the frailty, fractures, curved back and loss of height that are often regarded as a normal part of ageing. In fact, these are symptoms of a disease, osteoporosis, which can be prevented if steps are taken earlier in life. If allowed to progress without treatment, osteoporosis is one of the leading causes of suffering, disability and death in elderly people. Fortunately, there is now increasing awareness of osteoporosis, among both doctors and the public, and there have been important breakthroughs in its diagnosis and treatment.

Osteoporosis means porosity or thinning of the bones, whatever the cause, and is present in most very elderly people. Bone loss with ageing is a universal phenomenon but becomes a disease when bone mass falls to a level at which fracture is likely to occur. In normal young adults the bones are strong and only break when there is severe trauma, for example, in a car accident. With ageing and with certain diseases, the bones become thinner and, as a result, weaker so that they break much more easily. These fragility fractures are the hallmark of osteoporosis and are particularly common in the wrist, spine and hip.

The risk of having a fracture as a result of osteoporosis rises steeply with age. At the age of 80 years, one woman in three and one man in five can expect to have a hip fracture and a similar proportion will have spinal fractures. At the age of 50 years, a woman has a 40 per cent chance of having a fracture caused by osteoporosis during the rest of her life; the corresponding risk for a man is around 13 per cent. In the United Kingdom every year, there are about 250,000 fractures resulting from osteoporosis, of which 60,000 occur in the hip and 50,000 in the wrist.

Although most common in elderly women, osteoporosis can also affect men and may occur at any age from childhood onwards. The frequency of osteoporosis varies widely in different parts of the world, being particularly common in western Europe and the USA, and affecting white European and Asian populations more than black Americans.

As people all over the world are living longer, the number of elderly people in the population will increase dramatically over the next 50 years and this will lead to a doubling or more in the number of fractures resulting from osteoporosis.

The suffering and disability caused by fractures resulting from osteoporosis have created a major health problem in many elderly populations throughout the Western World; osteoporotic fractures are also an important cause of death in elderly people and 15–20 per cent of people who suffer hip fracture die within six months. The costs to our health services resulting from osteoporosis are enormous. It has been estimated that we spend £950 million each year treating patients with fractures resulting from osteoporosis and these costs

are likely to rise steeply as the numbers of elderly people increase.

CASE STUDY: FRED

Fred developed Crohn's disease, an inflammation of the bowel, when he was 16 and he required several operations to remove diseased intestine; he also needed steroid treatment. He presented with severe back pain at the age of 22, and an X-ray showed that the bones were thin and one of the bones in the spine (a vertebra) was crushed. A diagnosis of osteoporosis was made and he was given treatment to reduce the pain and to prevent further bone loss. In this case, osteoporosis was the result of a combination of steroids and reduced absorption of nutrients from the diseased bowel.

CASE STUDY: MARY

Mary was aged 56 years when she fractured her wrist. She had been well up to that time and had not experienced any previous fractures. The wrist fracture occurred when she tripped while out shopping and fell onto her outstretched hand. She was seen in the accident and emergency department of a local hospital and a plaster was applied to the arm. She was seen a few weeks later by an orthopaedic surgeon to check that the fracture was healing and referred to another department to have a bone density measurement made. The results of this showed that she had osteoporosis and she was advised to start hormone replacement therapy. In this case, no predisposing causes for osteoporosis were found and a diagnosis of postmenopausal osteoporosis was made.

CASE STUDY: CYNTHIA

Cynthia, aged 70, went to see her doctor because she noticed that she had lost several inches in height over the past year. She had also noticed that her spine had become rounded and that she had lost her figure – her abdomen seemed to have become much rounder and she had lost her waistline. Daily activities, such as housework and shopping, had become increasingly difficult as her back became very uncomfortable after standing for prolonged periods. Although she had generally been healthy in the past, she had experienced an early menopause at the age of 41 years, but she was not advised to take hormone replacement therapy at that time. X-rays showed osteoporosis of the spine. She was treated with physiotherapy and given medication to prevent any further bone loss. In this case, premature menopause is likely to have been a major factor in the development of severe spinal osteoporosis.

KEY POINTS

- ✓ Osteoporosis is the result of thinning of the bones, causing them to break more easily than normal

- ✓ Although most common in elderly women, osteoporosis also affects men and may occur at any age

- ✓ By the age of 80 years, one woman in three and one man in five can expect to have a fracture as a result of osteoporosis

How does osteoporosis develop?

NORMAL BONE STRUCTURE

Normal bones are composed of a shell of compact or solid bone surrounding connecting plates and rods of bone (spongy bone) within which lie the bone marrow. The thickness of the outer shell of compact bone varies in different parts of the skeleton; for example, it is much greater in the skull and bones of the legs and arms than in the spine. Much of the strength of the skeleton is the result of compact bone but the spongy bone also makes an important contribution. Bone is actually made up mainly of a protein called collagen and bone mineral, which contains calcium.

Bone is a living tissue which needs to be constantly renewed to keep up its strength. All the time old bone is being broken down and replaced by new stronger bone. If this process, which takes place on the bone surface and is called bone remodelling, did not exist our skeleton would begin to suffer from fatigue damage while we were still young! There are two main types of cell in bone: the osteoclasts which destroy bone and the osteoblasts which make new bone. Both of these are formed in the bone marrow.

As we get older the osteoclasts become more active and the osteoblasts less active, so more bone is removed and less formed.

CHANGES IN BONE IN OSTEOPOROSIS

In osteoporosis, the amount of both compact and spongy bone is reduced. Thinning of the outer layer of compact bone greatly reduces its strength and increases the likelihood of fracture. As bone loss occurs in spongy bone, the thick

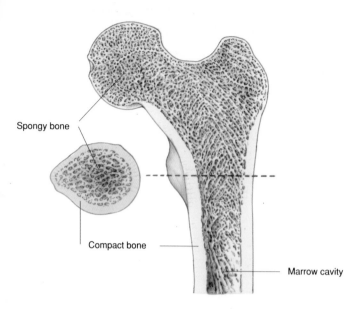

Cross and long section of bone (femur).

plates and rods become very thin and the continuity of structure is lost. These changes add to the weakening of the bones caused by thinning of the compact shell around the bone.

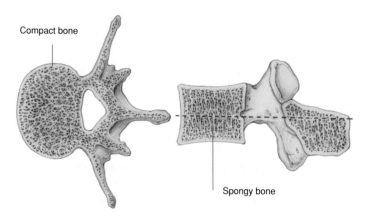

Cross and long section of typical vertebra.

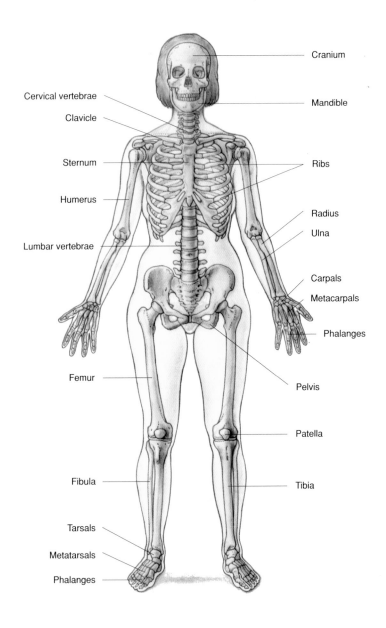

Cranium

Mandible

Cervical vertebrae

Clavicle

Sternum

Humerus

Lumbar vertebrae

Ribs

Radius

Ulna

Carpals

Metacarpals

Phalanges

Femur

Pelvis

Patella

Fibula

Tibia

Tarsals

Metatarsals

Phalanges

Front view of skeleton.

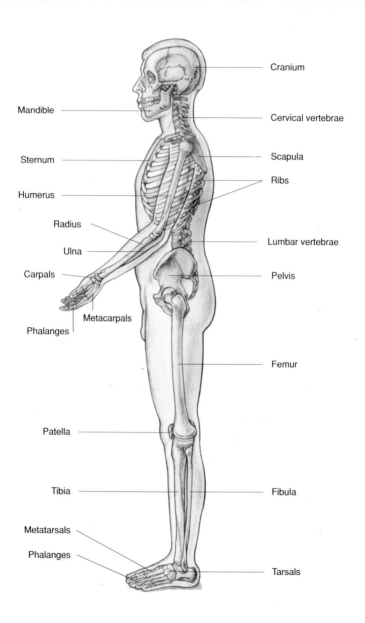

Cranium

Mandible

Cervical vertebrae

Sternum

Scapula

Humerus

Ribs

Radius

Ulna

Lumbar vertebrae

Carpals

Pelvis

Metacarpals

Phalanges

Femur

Patella

Tibia

Fibula

Metatarsals

Phalanges

Tarsals

Side view of skeleton.

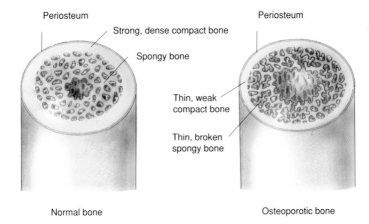

Periosteum

Strong, dense compact bone

Spongy bone

Periosteum

Thin, weak compact bone

Thin, broken spongy bone

Normal bone

Osteoporotic bone

Changes in osteoporotic bone.

BONE MASS CHANGES THROUGHOUT LIFE

Peak bone mass

During childhood and adolescence, the bones not only grow but also become more solid. By the age of about 25 years, the amount of bone in the skeleton has reached its maximum; this is known as the peak bone mass. Peak bone mass varies quite widely among individuals and is generally higher in men than in women. As would be expected, it is greater in those with a large body frame than in small, slim individuals.

The peak bone mass is very important in determining whether an individual is at risk from osteoporosis later in life. If it is low, then even small amounts of bone loss may result in fracture whereas, if it is high, an individual will be protected from osteoporosis. The factors that determine peak bone mass are not fully understood but there is a strong genetic influence, and calcium intake and physical exercise are also believed to be important. In addition, sex hormones can influence peak bone mass, for example, amenorrhoea (absence of menstrual periods) caused by anorexia nervosa or other illness will result in reduced peak bone mass, whereas there is some evidence that oral contraceptive use may result in a greater peak bone mass.

Age-related bone loss

In both men and women, age-related bone loss begins around

the age of 40 years and continues throughout life. In women about 35 per cent of compact bone and 50 per cent of spongy bone in the skeleton is lost during a lifetime, whereas men lose about two-thirds of this amount. The reason that women lose more bone than men is that, during the menopause, the rate of bone loss increases for a few years. As women have less bone to start with, lose increased amounts during the menopause and live longer than men, they are more at risk from osteoporosis. In fact, by the age of 80 years, nearly all women will have such a low bone mass that they are likely to have a fracture if they fall. The causes of age-related bone loss are not completely understood but oestrogen deficiency is known to be mainly responsible for menopausal bone loss in women.

In many individuals, age-related bone loss is sufficient to result in osteoporosis in old age. In some cases, however, other factors increase bone loss over and above that which would normally be expected during ageing. These are considered in the next chapter.

KEY POINTS

✓ Bone is composed mainly of protein and bone mineral, which contains calcium

✓ During childhood and adolescence, the amount of bone in the skeleton increases, reaching a maximum in the 20s

✓ From the age of around 40 years, the amount of bone in the skeleton starts to decrease in both women and men; this bone loss then continues throughout life

✓ The risk of developing osteoporosis depends on how much bone a person has as a young adult and how quickly she or he loses bone in later life

Who develops osteoporosis?

nyone may develop osteoporosis, but some people are more at risk than others. In any one individual, the risk of osteoporosis depends on a combination of factors including their age, sex and race. Thus an elderly woman is at much higher risk than a young man and Afro-Caribbeans are at much lower risk than Asians or white Europeans, regardless of age or sex. Genetic factors are important in determining peak bone mass and may also influence the rate of age-related bone loss.

Finally, in some cases bone loss caused by illness, drugs or lifestyle habits may greatly increase the risk of osteoporosis.

GENETIC FACTORS

As osteoporosis is so common, many people have seen its effects in one or more relatives and are concerned that they will inherit the disease. Osteoporosis is to some extent a result of ageing, but affects some people more than others. There is no doubt that there is some genetic influence in osteoporosis, although it is not so strong as in diseases such as cystic fibrosis or haemophilia. The peak bone mass is mostly genetically determined, but other factors become increasingly important in later years and may eventually determine whether or not osteoporosis develops.

Nevertheless, the risk of osteoporosis is increased in people with a very slight body build, which is generally an inherited characteristic. Also, it has been shown that women whose mother had a hip fracture in old age have twice the normal risk of suffering a hip fracture themselves.

STRONG RISK FACTORS FOR OSTEOPOROSIS

Premature menopause

The menopause is defined as the time when periods stop and usually occurs at about 50 years, although any age from 45 years onwards is considered normal. When the menopause occurs before this, either naturally or as a result of removal of the ovaries, irradiation or cancer chemotherapy, this is considered premature.

Women who have an early menopause are at high risk from osteoporosis and other consequences of oestrogen deficiency such as heart disease.

Amenorrhoea

Amenorrhoea (absence of menstrual periods) before the menopause may occur for a number of reasons. It is common in women with anorexia nervosa and in women who exercise very vigorously, for example, professional athletes, gymnasts and ballet dancers. Amenorrhoea also occurs in women who suffer from chronic diseases, for example, some forms of liver disease or inflammation of the bowel. In most of these cases normal menstrual periods have been experienced before amenorrhoea occurs (secondary amenorrhoea). Less commonly, disorders resulting from diseases of the reproductive system result in failure of the production of sex hormones at puberty, leading to delay in starting or complete absence of menstrual periods. Amenorrhoea is associated with low production of the sex hormone, oestrogen, and is a strong risk factor for osteoporosis.

Steroid therapy

Steroid therapy, usually in the form of oral prednisolone, is prescribed for many conditions including some rheumatic diseases, some lung diseases, inflammation of the bowel and some forms of cancer. Unfortunately, although steroids are very effective in the treatment of these conditions, they may cause rapid bone loss and lead to osteoporosis. It is not absolutely clear whether there is a 'safe' dose of prednisolone as far as the skeleton is concerned,

STRONG RISK FACTORS FOR OSTEOPOROSIS

- Premature menopause
- Amenorrhoea
- Steroid therapy
- Past history of fracture
- Thyroid disease
- Cancer
- Others, e.g. liver, bowel or kidney disease; some forms of cancer

but 5 milligrams daily or less is unlikely to be harmful.

Generally speaking, the higher the dose of steroids the greater chance of developing osteoporosis and those taking steroids for long periods of time are also at greater risk; short courses of steroids do not have harmful effects on bone. Steroid creams and ointments applied to the skin, steroid injections into joints and steroid enemas are believed not to lead to bone loss. Inhaled steroids, which are widely used in asthma, may have small effects on bone but are unlikely to cause problems unless very high doses are used for years.

Past history of fracture

Individuals who have already had one or more osteoporotic fractures have a much higher risk of having fractures in the future. The reason for this is unclear, but it may reflect more fragile bone structure in those who fracture. This is particularly true for women with one or more spine fractures in whom the risk of further fractures increases about sevenfold. All women with previous fracture, particularly at the wrist or spine, should therefore be considered at high risk of having more fractures in the future.

Thyroid disease

Over-production of the hormone made by the thyroid gland, thyroxine, causes bone loss and may result in osteoporosis if not treated early enough. The same effect may occur if too much thyroxine is used to treat under-activity of the thyroid gland, so it is important that women who are receiving thyroxine should have regular blood tests to check that the dose is correct.

Cancer

Some forms of cancer are associated with rapid destruction of bone, leading to osteoporosis. One of the most common of these is myeloma, which is a malignancy of the bone marrow.

Other diseases

Several other diseases are associated with a high risk of osteoporosis. These include some forms of chronic liver disease, kidney failure and inflammation of the bowel.

LIFESTYLE RISK FACTORS

Many aspects of daily living can affect our bones, including diet, physical activity, alcohol use and tobacco smoking. Although the effect of these on bone mass and fracture risk is generally less than the strong risk factors described earlier, they are important because they can be modified to reduce the risk of osteoporosis.

- Dietary factors: calcium and vitamin D deficiency
- Alcohol
- Smoking
- Physical inactivity

Diet

There are many factors in the diet which affect the skeleton. A low calcium intake in childhood and adolescence may lead to lower peak bone mass and, later in life, inadequate calcium in the diet may increase bone loss. Vitamin D deficiency, which is often associated with calcium deficiency, causes softening of the bones (osteomalacia) and also increases bone loss and the risk of fracture. High intakes of protein, caffeine and salt may also increase the risk of osteoporosis.

Alcohol

Moderate amounts of alcohol, for example, 14 units weekly in women or 21 units weekly in men, do not appear to be harmful and may even have beneficial effects on bone mass.

However, consumption of excessive amounts of alcohol increases the risk of fracture partly because of reduced bone mass and partly because of the increased risk of falling.

Smoking

Women who smoke have an earlier menopause and lower oestrogen levels than non-smokers. In addition, tobacco is believed to have harmful effects on the cells which make bone (osteoblasts). For these reasons, women who smoke are at increased risk from osteoporosis.

Physical inactivity

Low levels of physical activity in childhood and adolescence may lead to reduced peak bone mass whereas immobilisation at any age leads to rapid bone loss. In elderly people, physical inactivity is often associated with reduced muscle strength and an increased risk of falling and fracture.

RISK FACTORS FOR FALLING

Virtually all hip and wrist fractures and some spine fractures occur after falling. With ageing, the frequency of falls increases and there are additional factors which may further increase the risk of falling and having a fracture. Some of these are hazards in the environment, for example, uneven paving stones or steps, loose carpet edges, etc. Others are directly related to the health of the individual, such as poor eyesight, dementia, physical disability resulting from diseases such as stroke or arthritis, poor balance and general muscle weakness.

Alcohol and medications such as sedatives or tranquillisers also increase the risk of falling. Not only do these factors make someone more likely to fall, but they reduce the normal protective responses to falling, for example, putting out a hand to break a fall or regaining balance after tripping. These risk factors for falling are particularly important in elderly people and, when present, greatly increase the risk of hip fracture.

KEY POINTS

✓ Anybody may develop osteoporosis, but the risk is greatest in elderly women, particularly Asians and white Europeans

✓ Some of the risk of developing osteoporosis is inherited

✓ Other factors, such as premature menopause, steroid treatment and anorexia nervosa, greatly increase the risk of osteoporosis

✓ Bone health is affected by several aspects of daily living, including diet, exercise, smoking and alcohol intake

✓ An increased risk of falling over, as a result of hazards in the environment or ill-health, greatly increases the likelihood of fracture in elderly people

Symptoms and signs of osteoporosis

Osteoporosis only causes symptoms when there is a fracture. It is important to realise that bone loss itself does not cause pain or other symptoms; backache, for example, cannot be blamed on low bone mass unless fracture is present. Fractures that result from osteoporosis cause pain and disability; in some cases, the symptoms from these fractures persist throughout life whereas in others they may eventually disappear or improve. Wrist, spine and hip fractures are most common, although fractures in other parts of the skeleton also occur, particularly the pelvis and humerus (upper arm).

WRIST FRACTURES

These are also known as Colles' fractures (after the Irish surgeon who first described them) and are most common in women aged 50–70 years. Typically, they occur after falling forwards from the upright position, the woman putting out her hand to break the fall. They most often affect the radius, one of the bones between the elbow and wrist, but are known as wrist fractures because they usually occur near the wrist joint.

Treatment of wrist fractures

Wrist fractures are painful and need treatment at a hospital, generally as an outpatient, although more elderly patients may need to stay in hospital. The fractured ends of the bone are sometimes displaced and have to be manipulated into place before a plaster is put on to keep the wrist still and help the broken bone to unite. Usually, the plaster is kept on for four to six weeks, during which only very limited use of the arm is possible.

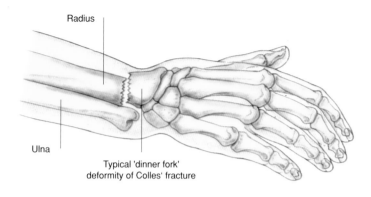

Radius

Ulna

Typical 'dinner fork'
deformity of Colles' fracture

Wrist fracture.

Long-term effects of wrist fractures

Although most people who have a wrist fracture eventually return to normal, several problems may arise during recovery. Sometimes the union of the two ends of fractured bone is not perfect, resulting in visible deformity of the wrist. About one-third of women have a condition called algodystrophy after the fracture, which causes pain and tenderness, swelling and stiffness of the hand, and may also affect the circulation to the area. In these patients, there is often persistent pain and stiffness which may last for several years.

SPINE (VERTEBRAL) FRACTURES

What is a vertebral fracture?

Osteoporotic spine fractures are different from other fractures, in that they do not involve the breaking of a bone but describe a change in the shape of the vertebrae, which are the individual bones that make up the spine. In the normal spine, the vertebrae are similar to bricks or a stack of boxes. In osteoporosis, bone loss may lead to crushing and compressing, and loss of thickness of the back, middle or front of the vertebrae or a combination of these.

The spine is divided into cervical, thoracic and lumbar regions containing eight, twelve and five vertebrae respectively. Only the thoracic and lumbar vertebrae are usually affected in osteoporosis, probably because they are subjected to greater weight-bearing than the cervical spine. The vertebrae most commonly affected by osteoporosis are those in the middle of the thoracic spine and the lower thoracic and upper lumbar vertebrae.

How do spine fractures occur?

In osteoporosis, spine fractures may result from falling but more commonly they occur spontaneously or as a result of activities such as coughing, lifting, bending or turning.

Symptoms of spine fractures

The symptoms caused by spine fractures vary greatly; in as many as two-thirds of cases there may be very little or no pain when fracture occurs, whereas others experience severe pain, although the reason for this difference is not known.

When present, the pain is usually felt in the back at the level of the affected vertebra and often spreads round at that level to the front of the body. It is often extremely severe and may remain so for days or weeks. In most cases, there is gradual improvement over months or even years; this is variable and, although some affected individuals become pain free after a few months, others may be left with lasting pain or discomfort.

As back pain is such a common symptom in the general population

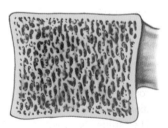

Normal vertebral body

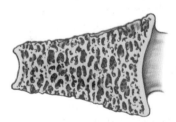

Wedging: loss of anterior or posterior height

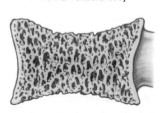

Biconcavity: loss of middle height

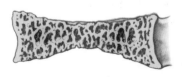

Compression or crushing: loss of anterior, middle and posterior height

Vertebral fracture.

and spinal fractures do not always cause pain, pain in someone with spinal fractures may be the result of other causes such as arthritis or disc problems, which are also very common. It can be difficult to be certain about the cause of pain in some patients, but a useful rule is that spine fractures resulting from osteoporosis do not cause sciatica (pain in the back which radiates down the leg); this is usually caused by disc problems.

Other effects of spine fractures

Spine fractures may also cause a number of other distressing symptoms. When several vertebrae are affected, there may be obvious loss of height, ranging from one or two inches to as much as six inches or even more. This height loss usually occurs over a period of years. This may be noticed by the patient because they cannot reach shelves which they had previously used or they appear to have grown shorter when compared with friends or family.

Height loss is often accompanied by curvature of the spine leading to the 'dowager's hump' or rounding of the back. This change in the shape of the spine causes the chest and abdomen to be pushed downwards, leading to protuberance of the abdomen, loss of the waistline and appearance of

horizontal skin creases across the abdomen.

The above changes cause severe physical and psychological problems. The combination of pain and spinal deformity often puts limitations on everyday activities such as shopping, housework, gardening and standing or sitting for long

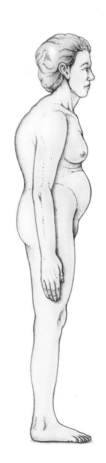

Dowager's hump.

periods of time. In very severe cases, the chest is pushed down so far that the lower ribs are in contact with the top of the pelvic bones, causing considerable discomfort. In addition, there is less room for the lungs to inflate and this may lead to shortness of breath, particularly on exercise. When the spine is very curved the sufferer often finds it difficult to hold the head up; attempts to do so may cause neck pain and headaches.

The change in body shape and its consequences result in loss of self-esteem and often affect social activities. As a result of the loss of waistline and prominence of the abdomen, many sufferers experience difficulties in finding clothes that fit them; hemlines tend to droop in the front and garments that are shaped at the waist can no longer be worn.

Many patients have a fear of falling which further restricts their physical and social activities; not surprisingly, depression is common in those affected by spinal osteoporosis.

HIP FRACTURES

What are hip fractures?
These are fractures of the top part of the femur or thigh bone. They occur

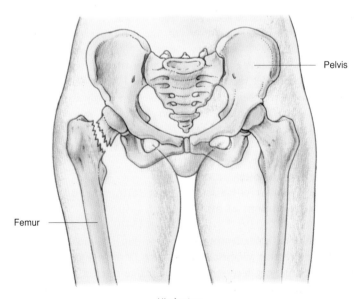

Pelvis

Femur

Hip fracture.

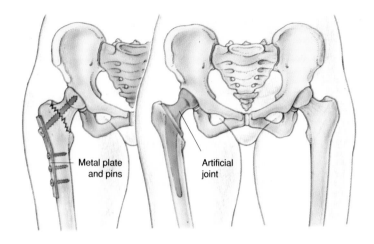

Surgical treatment of hip fractures.

most commonly in much older people, the average age of patients with hip fracture being 80 years. As elderly people tend to lean slightly backwards or sideways when they walk, they are especially likely to fall on the hip, particularly because they often fail to protect themselves by breaking the fall with their arms. Nearly all osteoporotic hip fractures occur after falling from standing height, although very rarely they may happen spontaneously.

Surgical treatment of hip fractures

Hip fractures are nearly always painful and require admission to hospital. Surgery is necessary to treat the fracture; if the ends of fractured bone are not displaced the usual treatment is to stabilise the fracture with a metal plate and pins but if the fracture is displaced (that is, the two broken ends are not lined up together), hip replacement with an artificial joint is often performed. As patients with hip fractures are elderly and often frail, complications of the operation are relatively common and most need to stay in hospital for three to four weeks.

Long-term consequences of hip fractures

About 15–20 per cent of patients die within six months of hip fracture. Of those who survive, only about one-quarter regain their former level of activity whereas one-third lose their independence, most of these requiring nursing home care. The remainder are more disabled than before the fracture and many require assistance with daily activities. Hip fractures thus have devastating consequences both for the patient and for families and friends.

KEY POINTS

✓ Osteoporosis causes symptoms only if a fracture has occurred

✓ Fractures of the wrist, spine and hip are particularly common in osteoporosis

✓ Fractures of the wrist and hip require hospital treatment; a surgical operation is necessary for almost all hip fractures

✓ Spinal fractures do not involve a break in the bone as other fractures do, but occur when there is compression of the individual bones (vertebrae) that make up the spine

✓ Spinal fractures may cause severe pain and lead to a height loss, curvature of the spine and other changes in body shape

Diagnosis of osteoporosis

MEASUREMENT OF BONE MASS

As osteoporosis is a preventable condition it is extremely important to make a diagnosis as soon as possible. In practice this means detecting low bone mass before a fracture has occurred. Until quite recently, this was not possible but there are now ways in which this can be achieved, using machines that measure bone mass – the amount of bone. These measurements are usually made in the parts of the skeleton where fracture is likely to occur, that is, the spine, hip and wrist.

The reason for measuring bone mass is that it provides information about the likelihood of fracture. Just as blood pressure is often used to predict the risk of stroke, or blood levels of cholesterol to predict the risk of heart disease, so the bone mass in an individual can be used to assess fracture risk.

How is bone mass measured?

There are several different methods which can be used to measure bone mass but the most widely used one is DXA (dual energy X-ray absorptiometry). This measures bone mass in the hip, spine, wrist or whole skeleton and is often called a bone scan. The value for bone mass produced by the measurement is known as the bone mineral density (BMD) and the general name for tests that measure bone density is bone densitometry.

The newest bone scan machines can make these measurements in only a few minutes, whereas older machines take around 20–30 minutes. Although X-rays are used in making the measurements, the radiation dose is very small, often less than the natural daily background radiation levels. Measurements can therefore be performed in children or pregnant

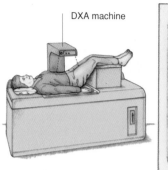

DXA machine

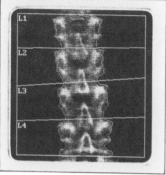

Monitor image
of lumbar spine

DXA imaging.

women if required, and can be repeated if necessary.

For measurements of bone mass by bone scan the person is required to lie on a couch. When bone mass is being measured in the spine, a rectangular cushion is placed beneath the thighs (this is done to straighten the lower part of the spine as much as possible during the measurement). A thin metal arm moves up and down over the site of measurement but there is no tunnel to pass through as there is in some types of scanning machines. There is no need to undress, although clothing containing metal objects may have to be removed before the scan. Finally, no injections or other unpleasant procedures are involved.

Another way in which bone mass may be measured is by ultrasound, using a method called broadband ultrasound attenuation (BUA). This is usually used for measurements in the heel bone (os calcis) and often involves submerging the foot in a water bath. It does not use any radiation and is therefore very safe. However, it is not so well tried as DXA and most experts believe that it needs to be tested further before it is used in clinical practice.

X-RAYS

X-rays, in a routine radiology department, are used to diagnose fractures in osteoporosis. They are not, however, very useful in detecting low bone mass because the density of the bones on an X-ray depend on a number of technical factors to do with the X-ray itself, as well as the actual amount of bone present.

It is thought that low bone mass can only be seen reliably on an X-ray when the bones have become half their normal density! Thin bones on an X-ray should therefore be taken seriously but, conversely, low bone mass will often not be detected on an X-ray.

At present, X-rays are the only widely available method for detecting spinal fractures. However, the latest DXA machines can produce very clear pictures of the spine and may eventually be used instead of X-rays to diagnose spinal fractures. One important advantage of this would be that the radiation dose involved is much lower for DXA than with ordinary X-rays.

BLOOD AND URINE TESTS

Osteoporosis cannot be diagnosed by blood and urine tests, but these are often used to look for other conditions that are associated with bone loss, for example, an overactive thyroid gland, liver disease or myeloma (malignant condition of the bone marrow). Blood and urine tests to measure bone breakdown and formation can also be used to measure rates of bone loss, but this is mainly a research procedure and is not widely used in clinical practice because they are not sufficiently accurate.

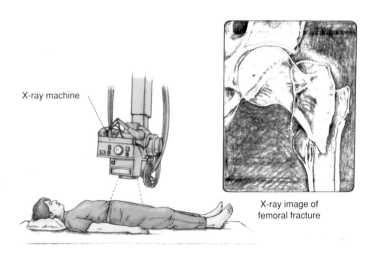

X-ray machine

X-ray image of femoral fracture

X-ray imaging.

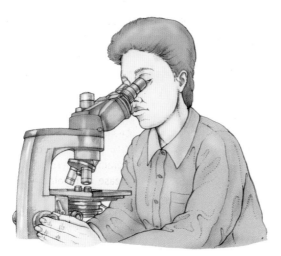

Blood and urine tests.

WHO SHOULD BE INVESTIGATED FOR OSTEOPOROSIS?

Screening for osteoporosis

At present, bone densitometry is the most accurate way of diagnosing osteoporosis. The question has often been raised as to whether all postmenopausal women should have bone density measurements.

At present, however, experts believe that there is not a place for mass screening for osteoporosis, either in postmenopausal women or in elderly people, although this may change in the future.

Use of risk factors to select for bone density measurements

In the absence of a screening programme, how can those at risk from osteoporosis be selected so that treatment is given before fracture occurs?

The method used by doctors at present is to select for testing people with strong risk factors for osteoporosis, for example, those receiving steroid therapy or those with amenorrhoea or an early menopause. All these should have a bone density measurement so that it can be established whether treatment is needed to protect the bones.

• **Use of bone density to confirm a diagnosis of osteoporosis**: Bone density measurements are also performed in people found to have signs suggestive of osteoporosis, for example, height loss or thin bones on X-ray, to ensure that a correct diagnosis is made.

• **Use of bone density to assess the effects of treatment:** In individuals who have already had one or more fractures, bone density measurements are often used to establish whether the fractures are the result of osteoporosis; sometimes, for example, in patients with many spontaneous spine fractures, this may be obvious but in some cases it can be hard to distinguish fragility fractures from those caused by trauma.

Finally, bone density measurements are used to assess the effectiveness of treatment given for osteoporosis. Most bone density units have a list of guidelines that indicate which patients should have bone density measurements.

• **Thinning of the bones on X-rays:** Doctors may sometimes comment that the bones appear 'thin' on an X-ray. Quite often this is a chance finding on an X-ray which has been performed for reasons unrelated to osteoporosis.

It should always be taken seriously because definite thinning of the bones on X-ray pictures usually means that there has already been considerable bone loss and the risk of fracture is therefore likely to be high.

WHEN BONE DENSITOMETRY SHOULD BE USED

Strong risk factors	Presence of signs suggesting osteoporosis
• Premature menopause • Amenorrhoea • Sex hormone deficiency in men • Steroid therapy • Overactive thyroid gland • Intestinal disease • Anorexia nervosa • Severe liver or kidney disease	• Thinning of bones on X-ray • Previous fracture resulting from minor injury • Height loss

Are bone density measurements widely available?

Unfortunately, bone density measurements are not as widely available as they should be and, in some parts of the UK, it is very difficult or even impossible for general practitioners and hospital doctors to obtain bone densitometry for their patients. This problem is now being addressed as a result of recommendations by the Department of Health, but it is likely to be some time before adequate services are uniformly available throughout the country. It is very important that bone density services are provided by experts, because running the machines, interpretation of the results and providing advice on treatment all require training and experience. The best units are generally based in hospitals and involve one or more consultant physicians with expertise in bone disease.

If bone density measurements are not available, doctors may have to base their decisions about treatment on the presence of risk factors. This is the best option in the circumstances but is far from ideal and is likely to result in unnecessary treatment for some people, because not everyone with a strong risk factor will actually have osteoporosis.

KEY POINTS

✓ The amount of bone (bone mass) can be measured in different parts of the skeleton; the most widely used method is DXA

✓ These bone scans can be used to predict the risk of fractures in an individual

✓ Ordinary X-rays are used to detect fractures, and blood and urine tests are performed to check for other illnesses that predispose to osteoporosis

✓ There is no screening programme available for osteoporosis in healthy women; however, bone scans are advised in people with strong risk factors, e.g. steroid treatment, sex hormone deficiency or a past history of fractures

Treatment of osteoporosis: general measures

GENERAL CONSIDERATIONS

Treatment of osteoporosis involves relief of pain, improving mobility, helping to cope with the psychosocial effects of the disease and preventing further bone loss so that the fracture risk is reduced. Although drug treatment is usually necessary to prevent bone loss, there are a number of self-help measures which can be taken by the patient to reduce progression of the disease.

Most people with osteoporosis find it helpful to learn about the disease and are reassured to find that much can be done, both to prevent further bone loss and fractures, and to treat existing symptoms. Knowing that there are measures that they can take themselves to improve their condition, such as exercise, changes in diet and avoiding falls, helps those who are affected to feel that they have some control over the disease and can improve their

chances of recovery. Many people also find it helpful to talk to other sufferers and to realise that they are not alone in having osteoporosis. Patient support groups, such as the National Osteoporosis Society, provide an important source of information about all aspects of the disease and supply a means by which patients can meet each other and professionals involved in the management of osteoporosis.

MANAGEMENT OF PAIN

How severe is pain in osteoporosis?

Pain is very variable in osteoporosis; some affected people have severe chronic pain whereas others have only minor discomfort. The pain that occurs after hip or wrist fracture usually improves rapidly after surgery, although pain-killers may be required for some time afterwards. In patients who develop algodystrophy after wrist fracture, physiotherapy may provide some pain relief and improve mobility. In very severe cases a procedure called sympathectomy may be advised, in which nerves supplying the affected arm are either cut by surgery or anaesthetised using drugs. Another treatment which has been used is transcutaneous electrical nerve stimulation (TENS), which is described in more detail on page 30.

Treatment of severe pain

In patients who have acute spinal fractures, the pain may be extremely severe and is difficult to treat. A period of bed rest may be necessary, although this should be restricted to as short a time as possible because immobilisation can itself directly cause further bone loss. Spinal corsets sometimes provide some relief, although most doctors discourage their use because they immobilise the spine and increase bone loss. Very strong pain-killers may be required in the early stages after fracture, for example, morphine-related drugs. Unfortunately these and other strong pain-killers often have side effects such as drowsiness, constipation and mental confusion and may also increase the risk of the patient falling once she becomes more active.

In those with severe pain that cannot be controlled by pain-killers, daily injections of a hormone called calcitonin is sometimes very effective. This hormone is produced by the thyroid gland (but is quite different from thyroxine) and has pain-relieving properties which can be very useful when other approaches have failed. Calcitonin is usually given by injection and, when used for the control of pain, is given daily or on alternate days for two to three weeks. It may cause side effects, particularly nausea and flushing when the injection is given, the nausea sometimes lasting for several hours. Vomiting and diarrhoea may also occur and there may be pain at the site of the injection. Nevertheless, worthwhile relief of pain is obtained in most patients, generally within a few days of starting the course of injections.

Pain-killing tablets

Once the pain starts to improve, many patients find that pain killers such as paracetamol or codeine, or combinations of these, such as Co-dydramol, Co-codamol or Co-proxamol, provide sufficient pain relief to enable daily activities to be resumed. In some cases, non-steroidal anti-inflammatory agents such as ibuprofen are effective. Individuals react differently to pain-killers, as far as both their effectiveness and their side effects are concerned, so it is worth trying different preparations if the one

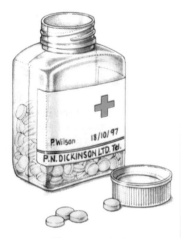

Management of pain.

a tingling sensation. The idea behind this is that the sensations produced by the machine 'block out' the pain caused by spinal fracture. Finally, attention to details such as comfortable chairs, with lumbar support cushions if needed, and a suitably firm bed are important and can improve daily quality of life.

PHYSIOTHERAPY AND HYDROTHERAPY

Physiotherapy, that is, the treatment of the symptoms of a disease by means of exercise, is very important

prescribed is not very effective. There are many different pain-killers available from the chemist or by prescription and it may take a while to find the best one, but it is worth persisting.

Other measures

A number of other measures may also provide pain relief. Heat pads, hot water bottles and icepacks may reduce pain. Some patients find that acupuncture is effective, although this is not generally available on the National Health Service. TENS (transcutaneous electrical nerve stimulation) also helps to relieve pain in some sufferers. This consists of a small machine that hooks onto a belt around the waist and contains small electrodes that are placed on the area affected by pain and cause

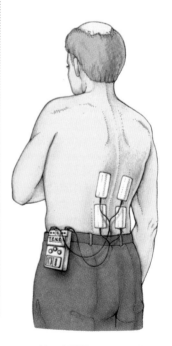

Use of TENS apparatus.

in the management of osteoporosis and is used to relieve pain and improve mobility. In patients with spinal fractures, the muscles around the spine often go into spasm as a result of the pain, and in doing so they actually cause more pain. Relief of this muscle spasm by gentle physiotherapy which relaxes the muscles will therefore help to reduce pain. Hydrotherapy (gentle exercise in warm water) also helps to relax the muscles.

Effects on confidence and risk of falling

Many patients with osteoporosis become very inactive, partly as a result of their pain but also because they lose confidence and are frightened that they will fall and have another fracture, or that exercise may lead to further damage of the bones in the spine. Physiotherapy and hydrotherapy can be very helpful in improving mobility and restoring confidence in such people. They also improve muscle strength and help people to protect themselves against injury if they do trip or fall.

Effects on posture

Another useful effect of physiotherapy is that it can improve posture. The presence of back pain and muscle spasm often makes the sufferer tend to round the shoulders and avoid straightening the back, but with gentle exercises and

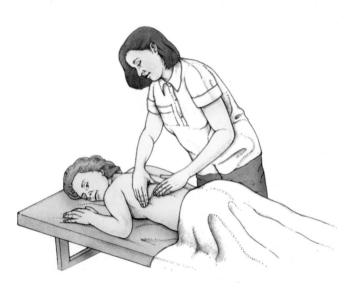

Physiotherapy.

relaxation of the spine muscles posture will often improve. Patients with spinal osteoporosis are understandably distressed by the change in the shape of their spine and the rounding of the back which occurs and it is important to realise that this can often be improved.

What exercises are best?

The amount and type of exercise which should be undertaken will vary according to how severely the individual is affected. Over-vigorous exercise can be harmful in some circumstances so it is best to seek advice, from either a doctor or physiotherapist, before starting exercises (see page 36).

In general, exercises that cause pain should be avoided although a little discomfort can be ignored. The National Osteoporosis Society has produced a booklet on exercises for osteoporosis sufferers which many patients find helpful.

KEY POINTS

✓ Pain can be very severe in osteoporosis and strong pain-killers may be necessary in the early stages after fracture

✓ Injections of a hormone called calcitonin often help to relieve severe pain after spinal fractures

✓ Other helpful measures include physiotherapy, hydrotherapy and TENS

Self-help measures

As mentioned earlier, there are a number of lifestyle factors that affect bone mass and for many of these an individual can take measures to improve the health of their bones. Many people find that by adopting self-help measures they feel more in control of the disease and are able to make their own contribution to improvement or recovery. These measures are just as important in people who do not have osteoporosis, because they will reduce the risk of developing the disease.

DIET

Calcium

A balanced diet is very important for the bones. In particular, an adequate calcium intake will help to achieve a good peak bone mass and will also reduce age-related bone loss later in life. Although many foods contain calcium, not all of these actually release much calcium into the body after they have been eaten and the best source of calcium in the diet is dairy produce, e.g. milk, eggs and cheese. Most experts believe that about one gram of calcium should be taken in the diet each day; one pint of milk contains about three-quarters of this amount (including skimmed milk, which actually contains a little more calcium than full cream or semi-skimmed milk). Unfortunately, some people are unable to tolerate dairy products and it may be necessary for them to have calcium supplements, because it is very difficult to manage to consume one gram of calcium each day without using dairy products.

There is a bewildering choice of calcium products on sale in health food shops and chemists. These contain different amounts of calcium and, in many instances, are insufficient to protect the bones against osteoporosis. It is therefore important to make sure that the

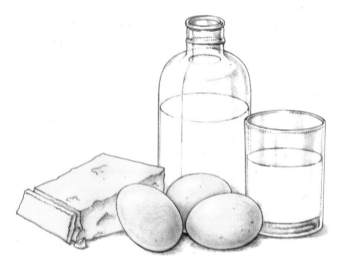

Calcium-rich foods.

preparation chosen contains enough calcium; if in doubt, it is best to ask the pharmacist or your general practitioner.

Harmful effects of excessive weight loss

Excessive slimming has harmful effects on the bones. Patients with anorexia nervosa often have severe osteoporosis, even though they are young, and although some of the bone loss is caused by amenor-rhoea, their low body weight also plays an important part. Anorexia nervosa often develops during adolescence, when the skeleton should be growing and bone loss at this stage leads to a low peak bone mass and greatly increased risk of osteoporosis. Conversely, people who are overweight tend to have a greater bone mass, but this does not mean that obesity should be encouraged, because it has so many harmful effects on health! The best course is to aim for a normal weight for height and body build; patients with osteoporosis who are under-weight should be encouraged to achieve normal weight if possible.

Are vegetarians at increased risk?

There are probably lots of other substances in the diet that are important for our bones. Other than taking plenty of calcium, however, special diets are not advised for patients with osteoporosis. Vegetarians are sometimes con-cerned that their diet may increase the risk of osteoporosis. Provided that they have an adequate calcium intake, there is no evidence that being a vegetarian is bad for bones; in fact, eating large amounts of protein, as in meat, may increase the loss of calcium from the body. However, vegetarians who avoid all dairy produce should be advised to take calcium supplements.

VITAMIN D

Deficiency of vitamin D is common in elderly people and can cause bone loss, so it is important to make sure that adequate vitamin D is provided. Vitamin D is made by the skin when exposed to sunlight, and even in the UK this usually provides enough to maintain normal body levels. However, in elderly people who are housebound or go out little or in Muslim women who dress traditionally, vitamin D deficiency often occurs. Vitamin D can be taken in the diet, but the main source is fatty fish such as halibut and mackerel, which many people do not eat regularly. Dairy products contain smaller amounts of vitamin D and a few foods are fortified with the vitamin. For those who do not go out of doors much, dietary intake is often insufficient and supplements are required.

Chemists and health food shops contain a large number of preparations containing vitamin D, often in combination with other vitamins and minerals. The amount of vitamin D contained in these preparations varies; the recommended daily

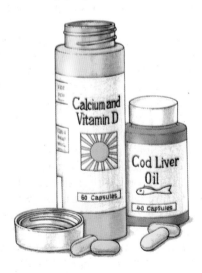

Vitamin D supplements.

intake is 400 international units (IU) but in the elderly, 800 IU daily is probably required. In these doses vitamin D is completely safe and has no side effects.

EXERCISE

Exercise is good for bones, as well as for many other aspects of our health. Complete immobilisation leads to rapid bone loss, whereas weight-bearing exercise can actually increase bone mass, particularly in childhood and adolescence.

In older people, exercise may slow down the bone loss which occurs with ageing and improve general fitness, thus reducing the risk of falling. So, from the point of view of preventing osteoporosis, it is advisable to take exercise at all ages.

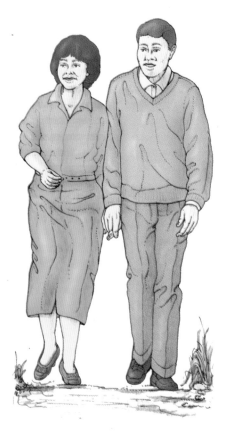

Exercise is good for bones.

What types of exercise are good for bones?

In order to benefit the bones, exercise must be weight-bearing and it will only affect those bones that are directly involved in taking the strain. It has been shown that jumping up and down or skipping can increase bone mass in the hip in young women and several studies have shown that brisk walking for 30 minutes or so for three or four days each week may reduce bone loss in the spine and hip in older women. Swimming, although good for relaxing tense muscles, does not benefit bone mass because it does not involve weight-bearing.

Over-exercising may be harmful

Very vigorous exercise can actually be harmful to bones, particularly in young women. Some marathon runners, ballet dancers and other sportswomen become amenorrhoeic as a result of excessive exercise and suffer bone loss and fractures. In general, it is best to take moderate exercise and aim for brisk walking for 30 minutes or so on as many days as possible. Use stairs rather than the lift or escalator and only use the car when strictly necessary!

SMOKING

Smoking is bad for virtually every aspect of health and the bones are no exception. There is also evidence that some treatments for osteoporosis may be less effective in those who smoke than in non-smokers.

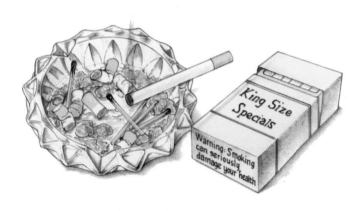

ALCOHOL

Drinking large amounts of alcohol may be harmful to the bones but the good news is that moderate amounts (e.g. 14 units weekly for women and 21 units weekly for men) may actually be beneficial! One unit is equivalent to half a pint of beer, a glass of wine or a single measure of spirits and it is best to limit drinking to the above amounts.

AVOIDING FALLS

There are many hazards in the environment which increase the risk of falling and simply being aware of these will help to protect against a fall that could result in fracture. Icy pavements and roads, uneven pavement stones and steep steps are obvious examples where everybody should be careful, but especially those who have osteoporosis. Potential hazards in the home include loose carpets and rugs, slippery floors and loose flexes.

Poor eyesight also increases the risk of falling and can often be improved by a visit to the optician. For those with difficulty in balancing a stick may be helpful, particularly when outside the home.

IF IN DOUBT, SEEK ADVICE

If you are concerned that you may have osteoporosis or are at risk from developing the disease in the future, seek advice from your general practitioner. The earlier the

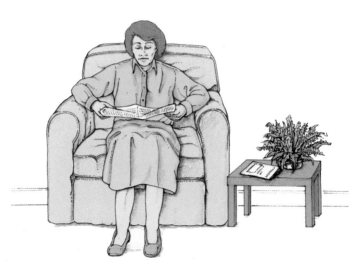

Support groups supply useful services, such as newsletters.

diagnosis is made, the better the outlook. Your doctor may refer you to a hospital specialist, because bone densitometers are usually based in hospitals. Alternatively, he or she may be able to reassure you that you are not at increased risk and put your mind at rest.

SUPPORT GROUPS

Many people with osteoporosis find it helpful to talk to other sufferers and in many parts of the country there are local support groups run by the National Osteoporosis Society (NOS). The NOS provides booklets on many aspects of osteoporosis which are written for sufferers and provide clear, practical advice. They also run a telephone helpline staffed by specialist osteoporosis nurses and produce a quarterly newsletter for their members.

KEY POINTS

✓ There are a number of measures that an individual can take to keep her bones in good health and thus reduce her risk of osteoporosis

✓ Diet is important, particularly calcium, which is available mainly in the form of milk and other dairy products; vitamin D deficiency should be avoided, particularly in elderly people

✓ Exercise is good for the bones at all stages of life

✓ Smoking increases the risk of osteoporosis; alcohol in moderation is not harmful

✓ Many measures can be taken to reduce the risk of falling and thus decrease the likelihood of fracture

Drugs used in treatment of osteoporosis: HRT

All the treatments currently licensed for osteoporosis act by preventing bone loss. They reduce the risk of fractures but cannot 'cure' osteoporosis, once this has developed, in the sense of restoring the bones to their previous state. This is why it is best to take steps as early as possible in people at risk from the disease. However, treatment is always worthwhile, even in people with severe osteoporosis because it will reduce the risk of having more fractures. No one with osteoporosis should be refused treatment.

TREATMENTS FOR OSTEOPOROSIS HAVE TO BE TAKEN FOR A LONG TIME

The drugs that are used to prevent bone loss act quite slowly and it is important to realise that they will not have immediate effects on existing symptoms, particularly pain. In addition, once spinal fractures have occurred, the shape of the affected vertebrae cannot be restored to normal so if the spine has become rounded this will not be corrected by the treatment.

All treatments for osteoporosis have to be taken for several years and, because there is no obvious effect on signs and symptoms of the disease, it may sometimes be tempting to stop taking the treatment or to take it only from time to time. This temptation should be firmly resisted because long-term treatment is required for a full effect on bone loss and fracture rate.

Depending on the treatment and on the availability of bone densitometry, many doctors advise repeat bone scans every one to two years to check that the treatment is working.

The rest of this chapter deals with hormone replacement therapy and other drugs are dealt in the next chapter on page 50.

HORMONE REPLACEMENT THERAPY

Hormone replacement therapy (HRT) has been used for many years in the prevention and treatment of osteoporosis. Studies have shown that it prevents bone loss during and after the menopause and reduces the risk of wrist, hip and spine fracture. Although mostly used in women around the time of the menopause, it is also effective in older women, in their 60s and 70s.

What is hormone replacement therapy?

The term 'hormone replacement therapy' refers to oestrogen alone or the combination of two hormones: oestrogen and progesterone. Both oestrogen and progesterone are produced by the ovaries and their levels decline during the menopause.

Although oestrogen replacement alone is effective in treating menopausal symptoms and preventing conditions such as osteoporosis and heart disease, it causes a small increase in risk of endometrial cancer, which affects the uterus or womb. This can be reduced by adding progesterone to the oestrogen for at least 12 days of each monthly cycle. The addition of progesterone prevents overgrowth of the lining of the womb, which results from oestrogens and may lead to cancer. It does not necessarily mean a monthly bleed, as

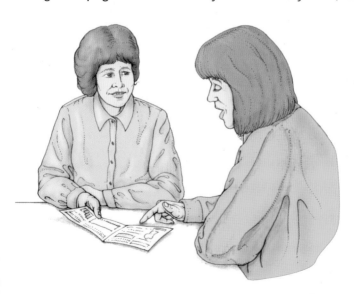

Doctor and patient.

discussed later. Usually, therefore, both hormones are given in hormone replacement therapy unless the womb has been removed (hysterectomy). The use of both hormones is referred to as combined HRT. In women who have had a hysterectomy, oestrogen alone or unopposed oestrogen is generally given.

The oestrogens used in HRT are natural oestrogens, in contrast to those used for contraceptive purposes, which are synthetic and more potent. As natural progesterone is difficult to take by mouth (it is broken down by the body when taken via this route) and has side effects, synthetic forms called progestogens are used for HRT. When combined HRT is used, the progestogen is usually given for 10–14 days of the 28-day cycle and oestrogen for 21 or 28 days (usually the latter). However, in some preparations both hormones are given throughout the cycle, in order to avoid regular withdrawal bleeding. These are known as continuous combined preparations.

What HRT preparations are suitable for preventing osteoporosis?

There are many different preparations that are suitable for preventing osteoporosis. These include tablets, skin patches and pellets that are implanted under the skin.

Tablets and patches are used for both oestrogen only and combined preparations, whereas the implants can only be used to give oestrogen and therefore are generally only used in women who have had a hysterectomy. Vaginal creams, gels and ointments are not absorbed into the body in sufficient amounts to protect the bones. The tablets, patches and implants all appear to be equally effective in preventing osteoporosis so a large choice is available. However, it is important to take a big enough dose of oestrogen to protect against osteoporosis; although this may vary a little between individuals, for most women the effective doses are:

0.625 milligram daily of
conjugated oestrogens
2 milligrams daily of oestradiol
50 micrograms (µg) daily of
transdermal oestradiol
50 milligrams of oestradiol
implant every six months.

Tablets are taken once daily, whereas the skin patches are applied once or twice weekly. Read the patient information leaflet contained within the medicine pack carefully and, if you have any questions, discuss them with a health care professional. You can also read the Family Doctor booklet *Understanding the Menopause & HRT*.

Short-term side effects of HRT

• **Vaginal bleeding**: Short-term side effects of HRT are troublesome rather than serious. The main problem for many women is the resumption of periods or 'withdrawal bleeds', particularly in older women who have not had periods for many years. It is likely that many women stop taking HRT for this reason. However, continuous combined preparations and a drug called tibolone do not cause regular withdrawal bleeds, although up to 30 per cent of women who take these preparations may have some irregular bleeding or spotting during the first few months. This is particularly likely to happen in women who are actually going through the menopause, so these preparations are only recommended in women who have not had a natural period for at least 12 months.

• **Other side effects**: Other side effects of HRT include breast

HRT PREPARATIONS THAT ARE SUITABLE FOR OSTEOPOROSIS PREVENTION

Combined oral
Climagest
Cyclo-Progynova
Elleste-Duet 2 mg
Femoston 2/20
Improvera
Menophase
Nuvelle
Premique cycle
Prempak-C
Tridestra
Trisequens

Continuous combined
Climesse
Kliofem
Premique
Tibolone

Unopposed oral oestrogen
Elleste-Solo
Harmogen
Hormonin
Premarin

Transdermal combined
Estracombi TTS
Estrapak-50
Femapak 80

Transdermal unopposed oestrogen
Estraderm TTS
Estraderm MX
Femseven
Fematrix 80

tenderness, feeling bloated, fluid retention, nausea, vomiting, headaches, indigestion and mood swings. When these do occur, they are often worse during the first few months of treatment and may wear off after that time. These side effects are particularly troublesome in older women and sometimes it is necessary to start off with small doses and gradually increase the dose over a few months. Although the list of side effects may appear rather formidable, it should be pointed out that most women feel better rather than worse on HRT, largely because of relief from menopausal symptoms such as hot flushes, night sweats and vaginal dryness. For those with troublesome side effects, skin patches are generally best because they release much smaller amounts of hormones into the bloodstream; alternatively, some women find that switching to another oral preparation is all that is required.

Although skin patches are generally well tolerated, they frequently cause skin irritation and occasionally more severe skin rashes may occur.

Long-term risks and benefits of HRT

When taken for a long period of time, HRT has both benefits and risks. These are still being studied and it is important to realise that we still do not have all the answers. However, a considerable amount of information is available and this should be discussed with your doctor before you embark on long-term HRT.

• Heart disease: The most important long-term benefit of HRT is its effect on coronary heart disease, **the most common cause of death in postmenopausal women.** Studies have shown that HRT reduces the risk of having a heart attack, possibly by as much as 50 per cent or one half. Most of these studies date back to the time when only unopposed oestrogen was used for HRT but there is recent evidence that combined HRT has similar protective effects.

It is not known how long treatment with HRT is required for this protective effect against heart disease; some of the beneficial effects on the circulation may appear quite quickly whereas others may take some years. Another important question that has not yet been resolved is whether the beneficial effects remain after HRT is stopped.

• Stroke: Although some studies suggest that long-term HRT use may protect against stroke (which is usually caused by a blood clot in one of the blood vessels in the brain), the evidence is not as strong as for heart disease and in one recent large study no reduction in risk could be shown.

• **Alzheimer's disease**: Alzheimer's disease is a distressing and relatively common disorder which causes dementia. In a recent study, women who had taken HRT were found to be less likely to develop Alzheimer's disease than those who had never had HRT. The results of this study suggested that HRT may postpone rather than prevent the onset of this disease, so that those at risk who took HRT would develop symptoms later than if they had never taken HRT. Obviously, this could prove to be a very important benefit of HRT, but more studies are needed.

• **Endometrial cancer**: As mentioned earlier in this chapter, women with a womb (uterus) who take oestrogen alone have an increased risk of endometrial cancer. However, this can be reduced by the use of combined HRT (a very recent study suggests a small increase in risk of endometrial cancer in women on combined therapy). There is no evidence that HRT increases the risk of cancer of the cervix or ovaries.

• **Breast cancer:** Most studies indicate that there is an increase in the risk of breast cancer in women who take long-term HRT. The size of this increase is probably about 30 per cent; as breast cancer is a common disease this is a significant increase in risk for any individual. Present evidence suggests that the increase in risk is similar for women taking unopposed oestrogens or combined HRT.

In most studies the increase in risk of breast cancer appears after 5–10 years of treatment. In a recent large study, women who had been on HRT for five years were shown to be at increased risk, particularly if aged over 60 years.

Interestingly, only those women who were actually taking HRT seemed to be at increased risk of breast cancer and, once HRT was stopped, the risk of breast cancer returned to normal.

• **Venous thrombosis**: Venous thrombosis is a condition in which blood clots form in the veins, most commonly in the legs (deep vein thrombosis) and spread to the lungs (pulmonary embolism). It has been known for some time that this condition occurs more commonly in women who take the oral contraceptive pill but until very recently it was believed that there was no increase in risk in women who took HRT. However, several recent studies have shown a small increase in risk of venous thrombosis in women taking HRT. As venous thrombosis is a rare condition, this only slightly increases the risk for an individual taking HRT and most experts believe that it does not significantly affect the balance between risks and benefits of HRT.

When should HRT be started?

It is never too soon or too late to start HRT if you have osteoporosis. Some premenopausal women with osteoporosis are prescribed HRT and, at the other extreme, HRT has been used to treat osteoporosis in women in their 70s and 80s. Premenopausal women who take HRT should be warned that it is not effective as a contraceptive and, if they wish to be protected against conception, should be advised to take an oral contraceptive rather than HRT. The use of HRT in older women (those 10 or more years after the menopause) with osteoporosis is likely to decline because of the high frequency of side effects and the availability of non-hormonal treatments. Nevertheless, some older women with osteoporosis express a preference for HRT because of its other beneficial effects; in such cases it should be considered.

How long should treatment with HRT be given?

This is a very difficult question! The problem is that if you want to be protected against having fractures for the rest of your life, you may need to take HRT for all this time. Although more studies need to be done, it appears that the benefits of HRT on the skeleton begin to wear off some years after stopping treatment and it may even be that, when HRT is stopped, bone loss accelerates just as it does during the natural menopause.

Although some doctors will recommend life-long HRT after the menopause for women with or at risk from osteoporosis, many others are concerned about the increase in risk of breast cancer and may advise that treatment should be stopped after 5–10 years. This is less of a problem now that other, non-hormonal treatments for osteoporosis are available, so that a woman can be switched from HRT to another drug if required. Women who have had an early menopause are usually advised to continue taking HRT at least until the age of natural menopause, e.g. around 50 years.

WHO SHOULD NOT TAKE HRT?

There are a few situations in which HRT should not be taken. In women with endometrial or breast cancer, oestrogens may hasten the progress of the disease and HRT is generally avoided. If a post-menopausal woman has undiagnosed vaginal bleeding, HRT should not be given until the cause has been found and treated. Pregnancy is also a contraindication to HRT and if there is any doubt about whether lack of periods is the result of the menopause or pregnancy this should obviously be checked before starting HRT. In women with malignant melanoma, a condition in which skin moles become cancerous, HRT may sometimes cause progression of the disease and is therefore best avoided in this situation.

In some circumstances HRT should be used with caution and only when other effective treatments are not available. Conditions that predispose to venous thrombosis, for example, obesity, immobilisation, blood clotting disorders, phlebitis (inflammation of the veins) and a past history of venous thrombosis, may increase the risk of developing a thrombosis while on HRT. Transdermal HRT may be preferable in such cases because it is released directly into the bloodstream and bypasses the liver (and so avoids some of the side effects resulting from the effects of drugs on liver metabolism). Some

SITUATIONS IN WHICH HRT SHOULD NOT BE TAKEN

Conditions in which HRT should never be taken
- Cancer of the breast or womb
- Pregnancy and lactation
- Undiagnosed vaginal bleeding
- Malignant melanoma (skin cancer)

Conditions in which HRT should be used with caution
- Endometriosis
- Fibroids
- Inflammation of the veins (phlebitis)
- Past history of venous thrombosis
- Severe liver disease
- High blood pressure
- Otosclerosis
- Migraine

gynaecological diseases, particularly endometriosis (inflammation of the lining of the womb, sometimes found in other organs outside the womb) and fibroids (non-malignant lumps of tissue in the womb), may become worse with HRT and occasionally high blood pressure becomes difficult to control when HRT is taken. In patients with severe liver disease, HRT may lead to worsening of liver function and HRT can also aggravate gallstones. Transdermal preparations should be used if liver disease or gallstones are known to be present. Otosclerosis – caused by hardening of bones in the ear and affecting hearing – may become worse while taking HRT. Women who suffer from migraine sometimes find that their attacks become more frequent and severe when they take HRT.

Balancing the risks and benefits

The decision whether or not to take HRT can be difficult and will depend on a number of factors. If it is taken for menopausal symptoms, 2–3 years' treatment is often sufficient and concerns about long-term risks and benefits are largely irrelevant. When taken for longer periods of time to prevent osteoporosis the balance between risks and benefits will vary between individuals and should be carefully discussed with a doctor. Although in general the benefits of HRT outweigh its risks, the fear of breast cancer is such that many women will be reluctant to take HRT for more than five years or so and, if bone protection is still required after that time, will choose to change to a non-hormonal treatment. However, others who have osteoporosis may accept the increased risk of breast cancer, particularly in view of the additional benefits for heart disease and may choose to continue HRT for many years.

• **Family history**: Women who have a family history of breast cancer are often particularly concerned about the effects of HRT. Breast cancer is a common disease and it is therefore not unusual to have one relative who has been affected, but this does not mean that the increase in risk of breast cancer with HRT is any greater than in a woman with no family history. If, however, there is a strong family history with several affected relatives, expert advice should be taken before starting HRT. Women who have a history of benign (non-malignant) breast lumps are not believed to be at greater risk than usual of developing breast cancer on HRT.

• **Conditions in which HRT may be safely taken**: HRT does not have significant effects on blood sugar and can be safely taken by diabetics.

Similarly, there is no reason why people with epilepsy should not take HRT, although some anti-epileptic medications may increase the dose of HRT required.

• **Should HRT be stopped before and during surgery?:** There is some disagreement among doctors as to whether HRT should be stopped before surgical operations. Some believe that it is unnecessary whereas others advise that HRT should not be taken before and for a few weeks after surgery. The decision will depend to some extent on the nature of the surgery and whether any risk factors for venous thrombosis are present in the patient.

KEY POINTS

✓ HRT prevents bone loss and reduces the risk of fracture in postmenopausal women

✓ Except in women who have had a hysterectomy, HRT is given in the form of two hormones: oestrogen and a progestogen

✓ HRT may be taken by mouth, as a skin patch or as an implant under the skin

✓ Side effects of HRT include vaginal bleeding, breast tenderness, nausea and fluid retention

✓ Long-term HRT reduces the risk of coronary heart disease and possibly also of Alzheimer's disease; however, it is associated with increased risk of breast cancer and venous thrombosis

✓ Life-long HRT after the menopause is probably required to maintain maximum protection against osteoporosis; alternatively, treatment may be changed to a non-hormonal drug after 5–10 years of HRT

Non-HRT treatments of osteoporosis

BISPHOSPHONATES

The bisphosphonates are a group of synthetic drugs which are increasingly used in the treatment of osteoporosis. Their main effect is to inactivate the bone-destroying cells, osteoclasts, thus preventing bone loss. Two bisphosphonates are available for treatment of osteoporosis at present, but in the next few years several new ones are likely to appear.

Etidronate

Etidronate was the first bisphosphonate to be used for the treat-

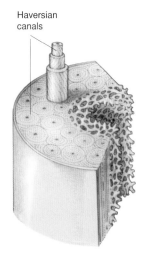

Haversian canals

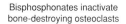

Bisphosphonates inactivate bone-destroying osteoclasts

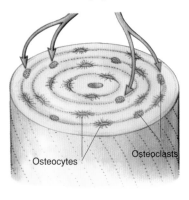

Osteocytes

Osteoclasts

Action of bisphosphonates.

ment of osteoporosis. It is taken in a 90-day cycle with calcium as Didronel PMO (the PMO stands for postmenopausal osteoporosis). The etidronate is given intermittently, two weeks' treatment being followed by 76 days (nearly 11 weeks) of calcium supplements without any etidronate. This cycle of about three months in all is repeated for a minimum of three years and usually longer. Etidronate is taken as a tablet once daily for two weeks of each cycle and the calcium supplement is provided in the form of tablets which are dissolved in water to make a fizzy drink.

• **Side effects**: Didronel PMO is very safe and has few side effects. Nausea and diarrhoea sometimes occur and skin rashes have been reported. Some people do not like the taste of the calcium supplement, but this can be changed to another preparation of calcium if required. As etidronate is absorbed from the intestine into the bloodstream in only very small amounts, it should be taken on an empty stomach at least two hours after the last meal and food should be avoided for the next two hours. It should be taken with a glass of water (not with drinks containing milk, as this prevents it from being absorbed into the body). Antacids, iron tablets and mineral supplements including calcium should also be avoided during the two hours before and after taking etidronate, as they interfere with its absorption. Most people find it most convenient to take etidronate at night, just before bedtime. The calcium supplement is taken once daily and may be taken at any time of the day.

• **Who should not take it?**: Etidronate should not be taken by women who are pregnant or breast-feeding, or if kidney function is abnormal.

Alendronate

Alendronate (Fosamax) is also a bisphosphonate and acts in a similar way to etidronate. It has been shown to protect against osteoporosis and is taken as a tablet (10 milligrams) once daily. Unlike etidronate, it is not combined with a calcium supplement although, if the dietary intake of calcium is low, calcium supplements are advised.

• **Side effects**: Side effects with alendronate are rare but include diarrhoea, pain and bloating of the abdomen and symptoms involving the gullet or oesophagus. The last usually consist of heartburn or indigestion and in a few cases ulcers and inflammation of the oeso-phagus have been reported. It is very important to take the alendronate tablets correctly, according to the manufacturers' instructions, because this lowers the risk of oesophageal side effects. The tablets should be swallowed whole with a full glass of water on an empty stomach at least 30 minutes before breakfast (and any other tablets which the patient may also be taking); thereafter, the instructions are to stand or sit upright for at least 30 minutes and not to lie down until after eating breakfast. The tablets should not be taken at bedtime or before getting up in the morning.

• **Who should not take it?**: Alendronate should not be taken by women who are pregnant or breast-feeding and should also be avoided if the kidneys do not function normally. If there is a history of problems with swallowing or severe indigestion, alendronate should not be taken.

Which bisphosphonate is the best?

Didronel PMO and Fosamax are both effective treatments for osteoporosis. There is no convincing evidence that either is better.

Can bisphosphonates be used for prevention as well as treatment?

Recent research has shown that they are effective in prevention as well as treatment of osteoporosis and they are therefore likely to be more widely used as preventive agents in the near future.

For how long should bisphosphonates be given?

Didronel PMO and Fosamax should be given for a minimum of three years. As bisphosphonates are absorbed into bone, they tend to stay there for long periods and may go on affecting bone for some time after the tablets are stopped. Most doctors believe that between three and five years' treatment should be given in the first instance. Bone density can be monitored after treatment is stopped and further courses of treatment given as and when required.

Are bisphosphonates alternatives to HRT?

Bisphosphonates are not hormones and therefore have no effect on menopausal symptoms or other diseases such as heart disease and breast cancer. The decision about which treatment to have will depend on a number of factors including the presence or absence of menopausal symptoms and the individual's risk of heart disease and breast cancer. In perimenopausal women (that is, in women around the time of menopause) at risk of osteoporosis, HRT is generally regarded as the treatment of choice but, if a decision is taken to stop HRT after 5–10 years and the individual is still at risk, treatment may be changed to a bisphosphonate.

In older women who do not wish to take HRT and in those in whom it is contraindicated because of breast cancer or other problems, bisphosphonates are a useful alternative treatment for osteoporosis. There is no evidence that taking HRT and bisphosphonates together is any better for the bones than taking either on its own.

VITAMIN D

Vitamin D is very important for bone health. It increases the absorption of calcium from the intestine into the body and hence ensures that enough calcium gets into the skeleton, which contains 99 per cent of all the calcium in the body. Vitamin D also probably has direct effects on bone, stimulating the formation of the cells responsible for bone formation. There are two forms of the vitamin which have the same or similar effects: vitamin D_3 (cholecalciferol) which is made in the skin when exposed to sunlight and vitamin D_2 (ergocalciferol) which is available from the diet.

Deficiency of vitamin D is common in elderly people, particularly those who do not go outdoors much, and a recent study from France in elderly women has shown that vitamin D and calcium supplements can reduce fracture risk in the hip.

Many doctors thus advise vitamin D supplements for elderly and housebound people. These

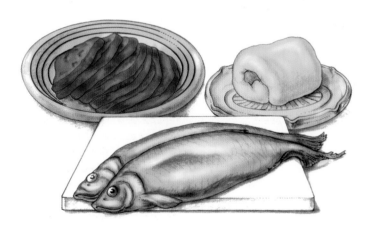

Dietary sources of vitamin D: liver, butter and fish.

supplements may be given on their own, with calcium or with other treatments for osteoporosis.

What vitamin D preparations are available?

Vitamin D may be taken by mouth or by injection. When taken as a tablet, the recommended dose is 800 international units (IU) daily. This may be taken in combination with a calcium supplement or without added calcium. For combined vitamin D and calcium supplements,

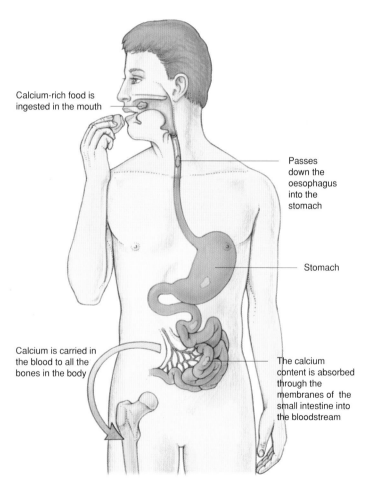

Calcium-rich food is ingested in the mouth

Passes down the oesophagus into the stomach

Stomach

Calcium is carried in the blood to all the bones in the body

The calcium content is absorbed through the membranes of the small intestine into the bloodstream

Absorption of calcium.

there are two preparations available which provide the right amount of vitamin D if taken twice daily. Cacit D_3 is provided as granules which are dissolved in water to make a fizzy drink; it contains 440 IU of vitamin D and 500 milligrams of calcium per dose. Calcichew D_3 Forte contains 400 IU of vitamin D and 500 milligrams of calcium per tablet. As its name implies, it is supplied in the form of a chewable tablet.

Alternatively Abidec and Dalivit, which are multivitamin preparations, each contain 400 IU of vitamin D per dose and will therefore supply sufficient vitamin D if taken twice daily. All these preparations can be bought from a pharmacist and no prescription is required.

Injections of vitamin D

Injections of vitamin D are also available and are usually given once or twice yearly. However, in some cases the uptake of vitamin D by the body after injection is low and oral treatment is therefore generally preferred.

Side effects of vitamin D preparations

In the doses described above, vitamin D is very safe. Occasionally

VITAMIN D PREPARATIONS

Preparation	Vitamin D (IU)	Calcium (mg)	Formulation
Abidec	400	None	Drops
Cacit D_3	440	500	Granules
Calcium and vitamin D	400	97	Tablets
Calcichew D_3 tablets	200	500	Chewable
Calcichew D_3 Forte tablets	400	500	Chewable
Dalivit	400	None	Tablets

Amounts are shown per tablet or dose.

the combined vitamin D and calcium preparations cause nausea, bowel upset (either diarrhoea or constipation) and flatulence. Vitamin D supplements are not advised in people who have high blood calcium levels, severe kidney disease or kidney stones.

Who should have vitamin D supplements?

Vitamin D is not licensed as a treatment for osteoporosis in its own right but is used, often with other treatments, to prevent vitamin D deficiency in those who are at risk, because it is known that vitamin D deficiency may increase bone loss, particularly in elderly people.

There are several groups of people at high risk of vitamin D deficiency; these include elderly and housebound people, some sections of the Asian community, those taking certain anti-epileptic medications, patients with liver or kidney disease, and people with intestinal malabsorption. Where necessary, it is possible to check for vitamin D deficiency with a blood test; if you are uncertain about whether or not to take supplements, it is best to seek advice from your GP.

Calcitriol

Vitamin D itself is not active and calcitriol is an active form of vitamin D. It has been shown to prevent bone loss and reduce the risk of spinal fractures and is given as a tablet (Rocaltrol) in a dose of 0.25 milligram daily. As it is very powerful, it may lead to high levels of calcium in the blood (hypercalcaemia) and urine (hypercalciuria) which can result in serious problems if not detected. It is therefore necessary to have regular blood checks when taking Rocaltrol, usually at one and three months after starting treatment and every six months after that. If high blood and urine levels do occur, treatment should be stopped and the calcium levels usually become normal within 1–2 weeks.

- **Side effects**: Symptoms of high blood levels of calcium include nausea, loss of appetite, vomiting, constipation or diarrhoea, thirst, passing more urine than usual, headaches and excessive tiredness. High levels of calcium in the urine may lead to the formation of kidney stones or deposits of calcium in the kidneys which may eventually result in kidney failure.

- **Who should take calcitriol?**: Most doctors believe that calcitriol should only be used in patients with osteoporosis who are unable to take either HRT or bisphosphonates. First, there is no evidence that calcitriol reduces the risk of hip or wrist fractures, whereas HRT and bisphosphonates have been shown to reduce fractures at the wrist, hip and spine. Second, the need for regular blood tests is seen by some patients and doctors as a disadvantage.

• **Who should not take calcitriol?:** Calcitriol should not be used in people with diseases that cause high blood levels of calcium or in women who are pregnant or breast-feeding. It should be used very cautiously if there is a history of kidney stones or evidence that the kidneys are not functioning normally.

• **Can calcitriol be used as a vitamin D supplement?:** No! Preparations containing vitamin D itself are much safer and provide adequate protection against vitamin D deficiency in healthy people.

CALCITONIN

Calcitonin is a hormone produced by the thyroid gland which inactivates the cells that destroy bone, thus preventing bone loss. It prevents bone loss in the spine but may be less effective in other parts of the skeleton such as the hip. Some studies have shown that it reduces fracture risk but not all experts are convinced and it is not widely used for the long-term treatment of osteoporosis.

Administration and side effects

Calcitonin has to be given by injection, three times weekly and is therefore normally only prescribed by hospital specialists. The preparation used is called Salcatonin (because it is made from salmon calcitonin). Side effects include nausea and flushing which occur shortly after the injection and are usually transient, although occasionally nausea persists for several hours. Diarrhoea, vomiting and pain at the site of the injection may also occur.

SODIUM FLUORIDE

This acts differently from the other treatments currently used as it increases bone formation and can lead to large increases in bone mass. Some studies suggest that it reduces fracture risk in the spine, but not all trials have shown these results and, if given in too high a dose, it may actually increase the number of fractures occurring in the hip; this is because high doses of fluoride can cause the formation of abnormal bone which is weak and more prone to fracture. Although it is licensed for the treatment of osteoporosis in many European countries, it does not have a licence in the UK.

However, it is used occasionally in this country by experts who can monitor the dose given and watch progress very closely. The correct dosage is between 15 and 25 milligrams of fluoride daily. These are much higher doses than those used to prevent dental decay in children.

Side effects

Nausea, vomiting and diarrhoea may occur with fluoride treatment and some patients complain of an unpleasant taste in the mouth. Occasionally, pains develop in the legs and feet; these can be severe and are sometimes associated with stress fractures.

ANABOLIC STEROIDS

Anabolic steroids are not the same as the steroids used to treat asthma, rheumatic complaints, bowel disease, etc. They are similar to the male sex hormone testosterone. Although they are licensed for the treatment of osteoporosis, anabolic steroids are rarely used because of their side effects. The licensed preparation, nandrolone decanoate (Deca-Durabolin), is given by injection every three weeks.

Side effects

Side effects include acne, fluid

CALCIUM SUPPLEMENTS

Calcium supplement	Dose (milligrams)	Formulation
Calcium gluconate	53	Tablet
Calcium lactate	39	Tablet
Cacit	500	Effervescent tablet
Calcichew	500	Chewable tablet
Calcidrink	1,000	Effervescent granules
Calcium-500	500	Tablet
Calcium-Sandoz	108	Syrup
Citrical	500	Granules
Ossopan	1,200	Tablet
Ostram	1,200	Powder
Sandocal	400	Effervescent tablets

Amounts of calcium are shown per tablet or dose.

retention, abnormal liver function and signs of virilisation including hoarseness of the voice and facial hair growth. Most experts believe that there is no longer any place for this treatment in patients with osteoporosis, because other safer alternatives are now available.

CALCIUM SUPPLEMENTS

Calcium is not regarded as a treatment for osteoporosis in its own right but is often used with other treatments to maximise their benefits.

A large variety of supplements are available, containing a large range of doses. The daily dose to aim for is between 1,000 and 1,500 milligrams (1–1.5 grams) for both men and women with osteoporosis; it is best to take these in divided doses three times daily, because a single very large dose of calcium is not very well absorbed from the intestine.

Do people with a good dietary intake of calcium need calcium supplements?

Obviously the need for supplements will depend on your dietary intake of calcium.

Many people find that they can achieve the recommended intake by small alterations in their diet and for most this is preferable to taking calcium supplements three times each day. A useful guide is that one pint of milk contains about 750 milligrams; if other dairy produce or calcium-containing foods are taken in addition to this amount of milk, calcium supplements are not necessary.

Side effects

Side effects from calcium supplements are rare. Some people find that certain preparations cause nausea or diarrhoea, but this can usually be resolved by changing to another calcium supplement.

RALOXIFENE

Raloxifene (Evista) is a new treatment which has recently become available for the prevention of spinal osteoporosis. It is taken as a tablet once daily. In some ways it acts like an oestrogen, but unlike oestrogen it does not cause vaginal bleeding or increase the risk of breast cancer. In fact there is evidence that it protects women against the development of breast cancer, at least for the first three years or so of treatment. Raloxifene does not help menopausal symptoms such as hot flushes and night sweats. At present it is unknown whether it has similar effects on heart disease to HRT or protects against Alzheimer's disease.

Side effects

Side effects with raloxifene are uncommon. However, it does cause a slight increase in hot flushes and may also cause leg cramps. Like HRT, it increases the risk of venous thrombosis and is best avoided in women who have had a previous episode of venous thrombosis or those who have risk factors such as phlebitis, immobility or obesity.

Who should not take raloxifene?

Raloxifene should not be taken by women who are pregnant or breast-feeding, or by women who have endometrial or breast cancer. Unexplained vaginal bleeding should be thoroughly investigated and treated before starting raloxifene. Raloxifene is not suitable for women with severe menopausal symptoms, as it may make these worse.

KEY POINTS

✓ Several non-hormone treatments for osteoporosis are now available, including etidronate, alendronate, vitamin D and calcitonin

✓ Etidronate and alendronate are taken by mouth; side effects are uncommon, although nausea, indigestion and diarrhoea may occur

✓ Vitamin D supplements may reduce the risk of hip fracture in elderly people; they may be taken by mouth or given as a once- or twice-weekly injection

✓ Calcitonin is sometimes used in the treatment of osteoporosis; it is given by injection, three times weekly

✓ Calcium supplements should be given with other treatments if the dietary calcium intake is low

Treatment of less common forms of osteoporosis

Most of the treatments licensed for osteoporosis in the UK have only been tested in postmenopausal women and, strictly speaking, are therefore only recommended in the prevention and treatment of post-menopausal osteoporosis. However, there are other causes of osteo-porosis which may affect children, premenopausal women and men.

STEROID-INDUCED OSTEOPOROSIS

One of the most common causes of osteoporosis other than postmeno-pausal osteoporosis is steroid-induced osteoporosis. There have been a number of studies recently that have investigated whether treatments used for postmeno-pausal osteoporosis are also effective in patients with steroid-induced osteoporosis. Although further studies are needed, it appears that bisphosphonates are effective in preventing bone loss

caused by steroids and etidronate has recently been licensed in the UK for this purpose. There is some evidence that HRT also protects against bone loss in post-menopausal women taking steroids.

In patients who need very high doses of steroids for three months or more, for example, 30 milligrams or more of oral prednisolone daily, some doctors believe that a bisphos-phonate should also be given to protect against bone loss. All patients who receive 7.5 milligrams or more of oral prednisolone daily for six months or more should, if possible, have a measurement of bone mass to see if they need treatment to prevent further bone loss. Women who are taking steroids should be advised to take HRT during their menopause.

OSTEOPOROSIS IN PREMENOPAUSAL WOMEN

Osteoporosis in premenopausal women may be caused by a number of conditions, including anorexia nervosa, over-exercising, secondary amenorrhoea and other gynaecological problems. Hormone replacement is often the treatment of choice in these women because they are known to have hormone deficiency. In this age group, hormones may be given in the form of an oral contraceptive or as HRT preparations. The choice depends partly on whether the patient wishes to avoid conception, because oral contraceptives are effective in this respect whereas HRT is not. Because the doses of hormones tend to be higher in oral contraceptives than in HRT preparations, patients who are very sensitive to the side effects of hormones often prefer HRT. Finally, the risk of venous thrombosis is probably greater with oral contraceptives than with HRT and this may affect the decision.

OSTEOPOROSIS IN MEN

For a long time it was thought that osteoporosis was a disease of women and that men were only rarely affected. Recently, it has become clear that osteoporosis affects men quite commonly and possible treatments are just starting to be investigated. Until the results of these studies are available, it is difficult to be certain about how best to treat osteoporosis in men and doctors have to use knowledge gained from studies in women, which is obviously far from ideal.

Deficiency of the sex hormone, testosterone, is sometimes found in men with osteoporosis. Testosterone has rather similar effects on bone to those of oestrogen and should therefore be replaced if deficiency is shown. It is usually given as an intramuscular injection, but may also be given in the form of a skin patch.

Bisphosphonates are also used in the treatment of osteoporosis in men; small studies suggest that they prevent bone loss although there is no information about their effects on fracture risk in men. Other treatments which have been used in men include sodium fluoride and calcitriol.

Vitamin D and calcium supplements should be given if required.

KEY POINTS

✓ Most treatments available for osteoporosis have been tested only in postmenopausal women

✓ Recently, etidronate has been licensed for prevention of steroid-induced osteoporosis

✓ Osteoporosis in premenopausal women is usually treated with hormones, either in the form of an oral contraceptive or as HRT

✓ Little is known about treatment of osteoporosis in men, although replacement with the sex hormone testosterone may be effective if deficiency is present

Questions and answers

Q: My mother suffered from osteoporosis in her seventies and eighties. Does that mean that I will inherit the condition?

A: Osteoporosis is a very common disease which affects one in three women by the age of eighty. It is therefore not unusual for someone to have one affected relative, particularly if that relative has lived to an old age and it does not mean that you will automatically inherit the condition. However, if your mother had a hip fracture in old age it means that you are at slightly increased risk from having osteoporosis later in life and you should have a measurement to check that your bone mass is normal. If your mother had osteoporosis of the spine, you do not need to have a bone mass measurement unless you have other risk factors for the disease. If you are uncertain, go and discuss with your GP whether you

should have any tests to check your bone mass.

Q: I have been told that I have osteoarthritis affecting my spine. Does this mean that I have osteoporosis?

A: No. Osteoarthritis is a completely different disease which affects the joints and is not associated with thinning of the bones. It can be distinguished from osteoporosis on a plain X-ray. Osteoarthritis is a very common condition which mainly affects the elderly and causes pain in the affected joints, including in the spine. There is some evidence that people with osteoarthritis are less likely to have osteoporosis and vice versa.

Q: Can the spine fractures which occur in osteoporosis damage the spinal nerves and cause weakness or paralysis?

A: No. Spinal fractures caused by osteoporosis hardly ever damage the spinal cord or the nerve roots. Back pain which radiates down one or both legs, with or without weakness and altered sensation, is much more likely to be the result of a prolapsed disc or some other cause.

Q: I have breast cancer and am being treated with tamoxifen, which I have been told competes with (antagonises) the actions of oestrogens. Does this mean that tamoxifen therapy will increase my risk of osteoporosis?

A: No. Tamoxifen is a very effective treatment for breast cancer and acts against oestrogen in the breast tissue. However, it acts rather like oestrogen in bone and protects against bone loss after the menopause, so that it is likely to reduce your risk of osteoporosis.

Q: My mother has severe osteoporosis with spinal fractures and height loss of several inches. Is it too late to give her any treatment?

A: No. It is never too late to treat osteoporosis, even in very advanced cases. Although there is no treatment which will cure the disease at this stage, there are drugs which will reduce the risk of further fractures in the future.

Q: Do I need to have regular check-ups when I am taking HRT?

A: Many GPs will see women on HRT at six monthly or yearly intervals for a general check-up. There is no need to have mammography any more frequently than the three-yearly screening routinely performed in the NHS for women between the ages of 50 and 65 years. If irregular vaginal bleeding occurs and persists after the first three months or so of HRT you should see your GP and may need to undergo a biopsy of the lining of the womb.

Q: How do I know if my treatment for osteoporosis is working?

A: There are no early signs to tell you if your treatment is working. Drugs given to prevent bone loss do not affect pain so don't expect any rapid improvement in pain or disability. Measurements of bone mass are the best way to show whether or not a treatment is effective but these are only sensitive enough to show changes after one to three years.

Glossary

algodystrophy: pain, swelling and stiffness which may affect the hand after a wrist fracture

amenorrhoea: absence of menstrual periods before the menopause

bone mineral density/bone density: the amount of bone or bone mass

bone scan: measurement of bone density

Colles' fracture: fracture of the lower end of the forearm, also called a wrist fracture

dowager's hump: curvature of the upper spin

DXA: dual energy X-ray absorptiometry; method used to measure bone density

endometrial cancer: cancer of the lining of the womb

fracture: a break in a bone

HRT: hormone replacement therapy

hydrotherapy: gentle exercise in warm water

hysterectomy: removal of the womb

menopause: cessation of menstrual periods

oestrogen: one of the female sex hormones

osteoblasts: cells that build new bone

osteoclasts: cells that break down bone

peak bone mass: the maximum bone mass achieved in young adulthood

physiotherapy: exercises to help the symptoms of a disease

progesterone: one of the female sex hormones

progestogens: hormones often used with oestrogen in HRT

TENS: transcutaneous electrical nerve stimulation

testosterone: the male sex hormone

vertebrae: the individual bones that make up the spine

Useful addresses

Amarant Trust
Sycamore House
5 Sycamore Street
London EC1Y 0SD
Tel: 0171 608 3222

Arthritis Research Campaign
Copeman House
St Mary's Court
St Mary's Gate
Chesterfield S41 7TD
Tel: 01246 558033

National Osteoporosis Society
PO Box 10
Radstock
Bath BA3 3YB
Tel: 01761 471771
Fax: 01761 471104
Helpline: 01761 472721

Osteoporosis 2000
47 Wilkinson Street
Sheffield S10 2GB
Helpline: 0114 2722000 (10–3, Mon–Fri)

Index

abdominal prominence **19**
Abidec **55**
acupuncture for pain **30**
age-related bone loss **8–9, 10**
alcohol
  – and osteoporosis **13, 38**
  – and falling **14**
alendronate **51–2**
algodystrophy **28–9, 66**
Alzheimer's disease and HRT **45**
Amarant Trust **68**
amenorrhoea **11, 66**
  – and bone mass **8**
anabolic steroids **58–9**
angina and HRT **44**
anorexia nervosa **11, 34**
    – and bone mass **8**
Arthritis Research Campaign **68**

back pain **17–18, 65**
beds, firm **30**
bisphosphonates **50–3, 61, 62**
bloatedness and HRT **44**
blood
  – calcium levels **56**
  – pressure and HRT **48**
  – tests **24**
body shape changes **19**
bone
  – cells **4**
  – changes in osteoporosis **4–5, 8**
  – densitometry **22**
  – density **66**
    – availability **26**
    – test for osteoporosis **25–6**
    – test for treatment effects **26**
    – see also bone mass
  – formation, sodium fluoride
    and **57**
  – fracture **66**
    – previous history **12**

  – X-rays **24, 26**
  – loss, age-related **8–9**
  – marrow **4**
    – myeloma tests **24**
  – mass, age-related loss **8–9**
    – changes **8–9**
    – measurement **22–7, 65**
    – peak **8, 66**
    – see also bone density
  – mineral density **4, 66**
    – measurement **22**
  – remodelling **4**
  – scans **22–4, 66**
    – HRT and **40**
  – softening **13**
  – structure, normal **4**
bowel inflammation and osteoporosis
    12
breast
  – cancer, and HRT **44, 46–7, 48**
    – tamoxifen and **65**
  – tenderness and HRT **43–4**
broadband ultrasound attenuation
(BUA) **23**

Cacit **55, 58**
caffeine intake and osteoporosis **13**
Calcichew **55, 58**
Calcidrink **58**
calcitonin **57**
  – for pain **29**
calcitriol **56, 62**
calcium
  – absorption **54**
  – in bone **4**
  – in diet **33–5**
  – with etidronate **51**
  – gluconate **58**
  – intake and bone mass **8, 13**
  – lactate **58**
  – supplements **58, 59, 62**

calcium (cond)
- with vitamin D **54–5**
Calcium–500 **58**
Calcium Sandoz **58**
cancer and osteoporosis **12**
chair, supports in **30**
cholecalciferol **52**
Citrical **58**
collagen **4**
Colles' fractures **15–16, 66**
compact bone **4, 5**
- changes in osteoporosis **8**
confidence, regaining **31**
contraception *see* oral contraceptives
corsets **29**

Dalivit **55**
death
- following hip fractures **20**
- related to osteoporosis **2**
depression in spinal osteoporosis **19**
diabetes and HRT **49**
diagnosis of osteoporosis **22–7**
Didronel PMO **51, 52**
diet
- to help osteoporosis **33–5**
- role in osteoporosis **13**
disease and amenorrhoea **11**
dowager's hump **18, 66**
drugs, risk of falling from **14**
dual energy X-ray absorptiometry
    (DXA)
- measurement of bone mass **22–3, 66**
- for spinal fractures **24**

endometrial fracture (cancer) **66**
- HRT and **41, 46–7**
endometriosis and HRT **48**
epilepsy and HRT **49**
ergocalciferol **52**
etidronate **50–1, 61**
exercise
- and amenorrhoea **11**
- and bone mass **8**
- for osteoporosis **31–2, 36–7**
- vigorous **37**
eyesight, poor **38**

falling
- avoiding **38**
- risk factors **13–14**
family history and HRT **48**
femur **5**
- fractures **19–21**
fibroids and HRT **48**
fluid retention and HRT **44**
Fosamax **51–2**
fracture *see* bone fracture
frequency of osteoporosis **2**

gallstones and HRT **48**

genetic effects
- in bone loss **10**
- in bone mass **8, 64**

headaches and HRT **44**
heart disease and HRT **44**
height loss **18**
helpline **39**
hip
- fractures **19–21**
    - genetics and **64**
    - sodium fluoride and **57**
- replacements **20**
hormone replacement therapy (HRT) **40–9, 66**
- balancing risks and benefits **48–9**
- check-ups **65**
- length of treatment **46**
- long-term risks and benefits **44–6**
- people at risk **46–8**
- in premenopausal
osteoporosis **62**
- short-term side effects **43–4**
- types **42, 43**
- when to start **46**
hydrotherapy for pain **30–1, 66**
hypercalcaemia **56**
hypercalciuria **56**
hysterectomy **66**
- HRT and **42**

implants, HRT **42**
inactivity and osteoporosis **13**
indigestion and HRT **44**
inheriting osteoporosis **8, 10, 64**

kidney failure and osteoporosis **12**

lifestyle risk factors **12–13**
liver disease
- and HRT **48**
- and osteoporosis **12**
- tests **24**

malabsorption of nutrients **2**
mammography **65**
melanoma and HRT **47**
men, osteoporosis in **62**
menopause **66**
- and bone mass **9**
migraine and HRT **48**
mood swings and HRT **44**
muscle
- spasm **31**
- strength **31**
myeloma
- and osteoporosis **12**
- tests **24**

National Osteoporosis Society **39, 68**
nausea and HRT **44**
newsletters **39**

non-steroidal anti-inflammatory agents
    for pain 29–30

oestrogen 66
    – deficiency and amenorrhoea 11
    – and bone mass 9
    – therapy in HRT 41, 42
    – combined 41
oral contraceptives
    – and bone mass 8
    – and HRT 44–5
    – for premenopausal
        osteoporosis 62
Ossopan 58
osteoarthrosis 64
osteoblasts 4, 66
    – smoking and 13
osteoclasts 4, 66
    – inactivation 50
osteomalacia 13
Osteoporosis 2000 68
Ostram 58
otosclerosis and HRT 48

pain
    – and bone mass 15
    – management 28–30
    – severity 28–9
    – in vertebral fractures 17
    – in wrist fractures 16
pain-killers 29–30
physiotherapy for pain 30–1, 66
plasters for wrist fractures 15
postmenopausal osteoporosis 2–3
posture
    – and osteoporosis 18–19
    – physiotherapy for 31–2
prednisolone 61
    – therapy and osteoporosis 11–12
pregnancy and HRT 47
premenopausal osteoporosis 3, 11,
    61–2
progesterone 67
    – in HRT 41–2
progestogen therapy in HRT 41, 42, 67
protein intake and osteoporosis 13

race and osteoporosis 2, 10
radial fracture 15
raloxifene 59–60
reproductive system disease and
    amenorrhoea 11
risk factors
    – for falling 13–14
    – for fracture 1
    – use to select for screening 25
    – for osteoporosis 10–14
Rocaltrol 56

Salcatonin 57
salt intake and osteoporosis 13
Sandocal 58

sciatica 18
screening for osteoporosis 25
self-help for osteoporosis 33–9
sex hormones and bone mass 8
sex-related bone loss 9, 10
skeleton 5
    – bone thickness 4
skin patch, HRT 42, 44
slimming effects and osteoporosis 34
smoking and osteoporosis 13, 37
sodium fluoride 57–8, 62
spine
    – corsets 29
    – fractures 16–19
        – pain management 29, 31
        – previous 12
        – sodium fluoride and 57
        – spinal nerves and 64–5
        – X-rays 24
    – osteoarthrosis 64
    – osteoporosis, genetic and 64
    – posture 31–2
spongy bone 4, 5
    – changes in osteoporosis 8
statistics of osteoporosis 1–2
steroids
    – anabolic 58–9
    – therapy and osteoporosis 2, 11–12,
        61
stroke and HRT 44–5
support groups 28, 39
surgery and HRT 49
swimming 37
sympathectomy 29
symptoms and signs of osteoporosis
    15–21

tablets, HRT 42
tamoxifen 65
testosterone 67
    – deficiency 62
thrombosis and HRT 45–6, 47–8
thyroid gland
    – disease and osteoporosis 12
    – tests 24
thyroxine overproduction 12
tibolone 43
transcutaneous electrical nerve
    stimulation (TENS) 29, 30, 67
treatment for osteoporosis
    – general 28–32
    – HRT 40–9
    – measurement of efficacy 65–6
    – non-HRT 50–60
    – self–help measures 33–9

ultrasound measurement of bone mass
    23
urine
    – calcium levels 56
    – tests 24

vaginal bleeding and HRT **43, 47, 65**
vegetarians and osteoporosis **34–5**
venous thrombosis and HRT **45–6, 47–8**
vertebra **5, 67**
– fractures **16–19**
vitamin D
– deficiency and osteoporosis **13, 34–6, 56**
– supplements **35–6, 53–7, 62**

vomiting and HRT **44**
waistline loss **19**
walking **37**
wrist fracture **15–16, 66**
– algodystrophy **28**
– previous **12**

X-rays
– for bone fractures **23–4**
– for bone thinning **26**